ALEXANDER
TECHNIQUE

ALTERNATIVE HEALTH

ALEXANDER TECHNIQUE

CHRIS STEVENS

ILLUSTRATED BY SHAUN WILLIAMS

An OPTIMA book

© Chris Stevens 1987

First published in 1987 by
Macdonald Optima, a division of
Macdonald & Co. (Publishers) Ltd

Reprinted 1988
Reprinted 1989
Reprinted 1990
Reprinted 1991

All rights reserved

No part of this publication may be reproduced,
stored in a retrieval system, or transmitted,
in any form or by any means without the prior
permission in writing of the publisher, nor be
otherwise circulated in any form of binding or
cover other than that in which it is published
and without a similar condition including this
condition being imposed on the subsequent
purchaser.

British Library Cataloguing in Publication Data
Stevens, Chris
    Alternative health: Alexander technique
    1. Alexander Technique
    I. Title
    613.7'8'0924   BF172
    ISBN 0-356-12430-4

Macdonald & Co. (Publishers) Ltd
165 Great Dover Street
London SE1 4YA

A member of Maxwell Macmillan
Publishing Corporation

Photoset in 11/13 pt Century Schoolbook by
🅰 Tek Art Limited, Croydon, Surrey

Made and printed in Great Britain by
The Guernsey Press Co. Ltd,
Guernsey, Channel Islands

To my mother

CONTENTS

Acknowledgements

With grateful thanks to my colleagues and students, especially Hanne Tietze for her careful criticism and to Walter Carrington for correcting my many errors.

FOREWORD

This charming little book invites everybody to join in an exciting adventure. Mostly, we are only too well aware of our problems in life but we don't realize just how we could help ourselves. We long for a helping hand, but we forget to look at the ends of our own arms.

F M Alexander, whose work this book is about, was a man with problems; but he was a great explorer, an explorer of his own capabilities, of his own potential, of himself. He found a practical way to overcome his difficulties; and if we follow his example we can rediscover some of his discoveries and they will prove to be as exciting for us as they were for him. Since I first met him, over fifty years ago, and he taught me his Technique, I have done my best to follow in his tracks and to help others to do the same; and the further I go, the more I realize just how far-reaching was his vision. New vistas of possibility open up all the time.

Chris Stevens has undertaken a similar journey and he describes some of the views of a new country that it has opened up for him. He has had a lot of experience in applying the Technique. He teaches it professionally and trains students to become teachers, but he is also involved in a programme of scientific research to make it more widely known and accepted. It is not an easy subject to write about because what it involves is so much a matter of subjective experience. How can the self-observation of mental and bodily habits, the exploration of our willing and wishing, our thoughts and feelings, be used as a reliable guide for gaining practical ends, still less to establish scientific truth?

The answer is that, if we can bring about evidently beneficial change within ourselves, although the means may be inevitably subjective, the practical results can be evaluated objectively.

To describe such a process to people who have neither had the experience themselves nor observed the results in others must be very difficult. It must involve a long stretch of the imagination. But in this book Chris Stevens has come close to achieving the impossible task. He has not quite managed to square the circle, but he has circled the square and shown us how to get round some of the rough, awkward corners of the problem. The result is a practical, useful, informative book, but above all, with Shaun Williams' amusing drawings, it is enjoyable and much to be recommended.

Walter Carrington, London 1987

INTRODUCTION

The Oscar winning actor, Paul Newman, the conductor,
Colin Davis and the authors, Roald Dahl and Edna
O'Brien have all spoken of the mental and physical
benefits Alexander Technique has brought into their
lives. It is also used by Sting to help him relax before a
concert, by Barry Tuckwell, the French horn virtuoso,
to monitor his body better in performances and by Howard
Paine to help him break the Commonwealth hammer
throw record. The Alexander Technique has helped
thousands of people from all walks of life. Here, in their
own words is what some of them have said about it:

Edward Maisel, Director of the American Physical
Fitness Research Institute writing on the effects of the
Alexander Technique
'There is an overall flexibility and tonic ease of movement,
greater freedom in the action of the eyes, less tension
in the jaws, more relaxation in the tongue and throat
and deeper breathing. There is also a sense of

EVEN HAMMER THROWERS CAN BENEFIT FROM USING THE ALEXANDER TECHNIQUE...

weightlessness and a diminution of the effort previously thought necessary to move one's limbs. Activity now becomes free and flowing, no longer jerky and heavy with strain.'

Dr Bent Ostergaard, Consultant Cardiologist, Aarhus University Hospital, Denmark
'The Alexander Technique is a realistic alternative to beta blockers in the control of stress-induced high blood pressure.'

British Medical Journal
'Alexander's work is of first class importance and investigation by the medical profession is imperative.'

Daniel Pevsner, Fellow of the British Horse Society
'The Alexander Technique removed a long standing back problem, improved my riding position and riding ability. Riders who take up the Technique always make a very significant improvement in their riding.'

Professor Raymond Dart, discoverer of the first
missing link between man and his ape-like ancestors,
Australopithicus
'The electronic facilities (of electromyography and
electroencephalography) have confirmed Alexander's
insights and authenticated the technique he discovered
in the 1890s of teaching both average and skilled adult
individuals to become aware of their wrong body use, how
to eliminate handicaps and thus achieve better (i.e.
increasingly skilled) use of themselves, both physically
and mentally.'

Paul Collins, Canadian National Marathon Champion
1949–52, Veterans' world record holder in 10 events from
200 kilometres to 6 days
'Through the Alexander Technique I was able to
rehabilitate my running after 25 years of being unable
to run through injuries, to the extent that I was able to
set ten world records for veterans in 1982.'

Professor George E. Coghill, anatomist and
physiologist
'Mr Alexander's method lays hold of the individual as a
whole, as a self-vitalizing agent. He reconditions and re-
educates the reflex mechanisms and brings their habits
into normal relation with the functioning of the organism
as a whole. I regard this method as thoroughly scientific
and educationally sound.'

Tony Buzan, inventor of Mind Maps, author of *Use Your
Head* and *The Evolving Brain*.
'The Alexander Technique transformed my life. It is the
result of an acknowledged genius. I would recommend
it to anyone.'

George Bernard Shaw, playwright
'Alexander established not only the beginnings of a far
reaching science of the apparently involuntary
movements we call reflexes, but a technique of correction
and self-control which forms a substantial addition to
our very slender resources in personal education.'

Professor John Dewey, educator and philosopher
'In the present state of the world it is evident that the
control we have gained of physical energies, heat, light,
electricity, etc, without first having secured control of
ourselves is a perilous affair. If there can be developed
a technique which will enable individuals really to secure
the right use of themselves, then the factor on which
depends the final use of all other forms of energy will
be brought under control. Mr Alexander has evolved this
technique.'

Sir Charles Sherrington, Nobel prizewinner for
physiology and medicine
'Mr Alexander has done a service to the subject by
insistently treating each act as involving the whole
integrated individual, the whole psychophysical man.
To take a step is an affair not of this or that limb solely

but of the total neuromuscular activity of the moment
– not least of the head and neck.'

John Cleese, comedian and actor
'I find the Alexander Technique very helpful in my work.
Things happen without you trying. They get to be light
and relaxed. You must get an Alexander teacher to show
it to you.'

Aldous Huxley, writing of the Alexander Technique
'It is now possible to conceive of a totally new type of
education affecting the entire range of human activity,
from the physiological, through the intellectual, moral
and practical, to the spiritual – an education which, by
teaching them the proper use of the self, would preserve
children and adults from most of the diseases and evil
habits that now afflict them.'

W H M Carrington, writing on the Alexander
Technique
'Our human upright posture is a unique accomplishment
. . . a most delicate balance, an equation of forces brought
about by an interplay of the sensory and motor
mechanisms, by which all muscular effort is practically
eliminated. The unique quality of the whole performance
lies in this reduction of effort.'

Professor Frank Pierce Jones, author of *Body
Awareness in Action: A Study of the Alexander
Technique*
'The Alexander Technique doesn't teach you something
to do. It teaches you how to bring more practical
intelligence into what you are already doing; how to
eliminate stereotyped responses; how to deal with habit
and change. It leaves you free to choose your own goal
but gives you a better use of yourself while you work
toward it . . . It opens a window onto the little known
area between stimulus and response and gives you the
self-knowledge you need in order to change the pattern

of your response – or, if you choose, not to make it at all.'

F M Alexander

'Every man, woman and child holds the possibility of physical perfection; it rests with each of us to attain it by personal understanding and effort.'

In this book I aim to explain why so many people have found the Alexander Technique helpful. In addition I want to communicate something of the process Alexander went through, not just because of historical interest, but because to learn the Technique each of us has to undertake a similar journey. Although a map is no substitute for real countryside, even a rough sketch map helps us to find our way in unknown terrain. I hope this guide will give you some views of a new country.

1. WHAT IS ALEXANDER TECHNIQUE?

In 1894 a young Australian actor began to teach a method for improving the way we use our bodies. His name was Frederick Matthias Alexander and his technique was soon being used by fellow actors. Later singers, dancers and musicians began to use it to improve their performance (today it is taught in leading drama and music colleges).

Some of his amateur colleagues were doctors and it quickly became obvious to them that, although the Technique was not a therapy, it did have therapeutic effects. These physicians, having tested the Technique on themselves, began sending some of their patients to Alexander. The first of these were people with breathing problems; since then the Technique has proved useful in a wide range of complaints.

As Dr Wilfred Barlow, a leading consultant in physical medicine at a London hospital reports, the Technqiue can also be used beneficially in stress-related diseases such as ulcers and other digestive disorders, some forms of heart disease and high blood pressure, asthma and chronic bronchitis, tension-related sexual disorders, epilepsy and migraine. He found it of particular use in the rehabilitation phase of many illnesses. The range of rheumatic disorders from disc lesions, low back pain, arthritis, to tennis elbow and frozen shoulders also respond well. In the area of mental health, Barlow reports that the Technique has had considerable success in helping patients suffering from anxiety and depression.

This combination of improvement of performance and better health was well summarized by Nobel Prizewinner for Medicine and Physiology, Professor Nikolaas Tinbergen in his acceptance speech, when he reported '. . .very striking improvements in such diverse things as high blood pressure, breathing, depth of sleep, overall cheerfulness and mental alertness, resilience against outside pressures, and also in such a refined skill as playing a stringed musical instrument'.

Alexander moved from Australia to London in 1904 with letters of introduction from a leading Australian surgeon to his colleagues in London. Some of the latter recognized the usefulness of his Technique and co-operated with Alexander until his death in 1955. This support continues today as we will see in more detail later.

ALEXANDER AND HIS DISCOVERY

Alexander was born in 1869 on the island of Tasmania. He grew up in the country and, although he started at the local school, bad health made it impossible for him to continue, and he was taught at home. Alexander developed a passion for Shakespeare and at an early age resolved to become an actor. He developed a repertoire of humorous monologues and Shakespearean speeches.

Throughout his early life, FM, as he was later to be called, suffered from poor health. He had been born prematurely and only survived due to his mother's ingenuity and persistence in finding a way to feed her

infant. His mother was a remarkable woman, who acted as the local midwife. Alexander told how he remembered that often, when responding to an urgent call, she would jump her horse over the farm fence, rather than wait to open the gate. Later, when FM was in London, she travelled from Australia to stay with him. One day, whilst crossing a road, she fell and her hand was run over by the wheel of a horse-drawn delivery van. This broke her wrist and damaged the nerves to her hand. Told she had lost the use of her hand, she practised directing her hand to move, and after months of effort she was successful and completely regained the use of her hand.

Although slight in build, Alexander inherited his mother's strength of character. He left home early in his teens, taking a job with the Mount Bishoff Tin Mining Company until he saved enough money to go to the Australian mainland. Once in Melbourne he took acting and elocution lessons, and eventually formed his own theatre company. However all was not well; as he gained recognition and had more frequent engagements, the stress told on his voice until, at one crucial performance, he was barely able to finish. He consulted doctors and voice teachers who suggested a rest cure. So for two weeks before his next big performance he tried resting his voice, not speaking at all for that time. On the night of the performance he was appalled to find that his problem had returned.

The next day, we are told, he went back to the doctor who had prescribed the rest cure and asked what he recommended now. More of the same was the reply. Alexander was not amused. He wanted to know the cause of the problem.

'Is it not fair, then,' he asked, 'to conclude that it was something I was doing that evening in using my voice that was the cause of the trouble?'

'Yes, that must be so,' replied the doctor.

'Can you tell me, then,' asked FM, 'what it was that I did that caused the trouble?' The doctor admitted that he could not.

'Very well,' said Alexander, 'if that is so, I must try and find out for myself.'

However this was easier said than done. He did have some clues to go on: firstly, he knew that the problem had something to do with what he did on stage as he did not have problems with his voice when he was not acting; secondly, his friends told him that when he was on stage he made a loud gasping sound as he breathed in between lines – you can hear this often today with singers, actors and public speakers, particularly when they are nervous.

ALEXANDER'S FRIENDS TOLD HIM THAT WHEN HE WAS ON STAGE HE MADE A LOUD GASPING SOUND...

Alexander decided to observe himself in a mirror, first when he spoke normally and then when he recited to see if he could detect any difference. He began to notice a pattern emerging. When he got ready to recite he drew in air with a noisy gasp, at about the same time he tensed his neck muscles which pulled his head back and down. He also found that this made him compress his vocal cords. Finally he noticed that he had made his whole body shorter and tenser, restricting his breathing and general freedom of movement. When he looked again at his normal speaking, he found the same tendencies, just less so.

By means of careful experiment Alexander found a way of preventing the pattern from starting. He did this by not allowing himself to 'get ready' in his habitual way. He then made use of his observations to find new and better ways of using the various parts of his body involved in reciting. The result was, that after a long period of practice, his voice problem disappeared. Quite unexpectedly, Alexander also noted a dramatic improvement in his general health.

HOW IS ALEXANDER'S DISCOVERY RELEVANT?

After Alexander had made his discovery, the improvement in his performance was so noticeable that people asked him what he had done. As he showed them, it soon became clear that many of them also suffered from the same general problem. Originally Alexander had thought that the problem only applied to him, but his observations and discussions soon led him to believe that the problem was a very common one indeed.

To show people what he meant about the way they held their bodies, he had to get them to observe themselves, much as he had done in the mirror. Because this was difficult (it had taken Alexander several years to make his discovery), he quickly learnt to guide people's movements with his hands.

Today most teachers of the Alexander Technique use the same method. Starting with simple actions, such as sitting, standing, walking and lying down, the teacher and student work together to pinpoint the ways in which the student habitually uses his body incorrectly.

With the practical help of the teacher the student can learn how to stop such harmful habits. This is usually done through a combination of demonstration, verbal

PUTTING THE HEAD BACK AND DOWN AND SHORTENING THE BODY WHEN UNDER STRESS.

THE RESULT OF 'GIVING DIRECTIONS'.

instructions and gentle guidance with the hands. The latter is especially important to give the student a reliable experience of what it actually feels like to use his body correctly. As a result the student learns how to let the body work in a freer and more natural way. Once this has become established it is possible to apply the principles to more complex and demanding situations.

As they progress students often realize how their specific problems or symptoms were caused by the general misuse of their bodies. My own experience may make this clearer.

I first took Alexander lessons because of persistent back pain. I had tried conventional medical treatment, osteopathy and yoga. All gave short-term relief but the pain kept coming back. When I went for lessons in the

Alexander Technique my specific symptoms were largely ignored by my teacher. Instead I was helped to recognize and prevent the habitual way I stiffened my body. As I began to 'leave my body alone', my back pain lessened and eventually virtually disappeared. Perhaps even more important was learning how I had caused the problem myself and how I could take responsibility for my own wellbeing.

As with many other things the roots of my problem were in my childhood. I can remember having back pain when I was eight years old (incidentally I was recently surprised to find that this is not at all unusual). Photographs of that time show me developing a tilt of my head to one side. In adolescence I grew very quickly and remember clearly never being able to sit comfortably in school chairs. By the time I reached university, my back problem was a chronic one.

With the help of my Alexander teacher I discovered that I slumped badly when I sat down, with tight and short belly muscles pulling down on my ribs and spine, forcing my head and shoulders forward, which in turn caused my neck, shoulder and back muscles to be under considerable strain. I learnt gradually how to let go of the shortening of the belly muscles by directing them to release, a sensation my teacher was able to help me actually experience through the skilful use of his hands. The result – I slumped less and my breathing was easier because the ribs could move more freely; my head balance improved as he helped me to release the excessive tension and shortness in my neck muscles; similarly, my shoulders, which had always been very rounded, began to broaden and take up a naturally straighter position; and I gained an inch in height and broadened around my chest as well as my shoulders – to the extent that after a while my shirts and jackets became too small for me.

My own experience underlines the fact that the Alexander Technique is not a therapy. Instead I was learning how to allow my whole body to work in an

unrestricted, more natural way. In my case, certain symptoms were cleared up as I learnt the Technique, but such 'cures' are incidental and the usefulness of the Technique is in no way dependent on them. (In fact, as I have learnt in my research, there are many causes of back pain that are not related to body use, and any prospective student who suffers from back pain should be aware of this fact.) However, as I discovered for myself, there are other, even more important, reasons for learning the Technique. Firstly, I found I was more competent in my chosen activities, lecturing and practising yoga. Secondly, I found I had much more energy and took up running and swimming, activities I had dropped when I left school, and was excited and stimulated to discover I could do these activities better than when I was a teenager. At the same time I was able to think more clearly and went back into academic life, researching into the Technique.

Having said this, I am pleased to report that I still have my problems and am by no means perfect. However the Technique has given me a set of practical tools with which to tackle difficulties and make the most of my talents. What is even more exciting is there appears to be no end to the process. Each new discovery illuminates a new possibility, giving the potential for continuing and self-sustaining growth.

WHAT KINDS OF PEOPLE FIND THE TECHNIQUE USEFUL?

Jane H is a pianist of many years experience. She had had a successful concert career and taught in a conservatoire. However, she confided to me, she had a problem with her playing. A particular piece required a long and fast arm movement to reach a high note. She had spent a great deal of time trying to improve her technique, but the sound of the note remained unsatisfactory.

1. WHAT IS ALEXANDER TECHNIQUE?

She demonstrated the piece for me and it soon became clear that before she began to move her arm she was tightening her neck and hunching her shoulders just enough to affect the movement but not enough to be noticed by the casual observer. I was able to alert Jane to this muscle tensing and show her how to stop it happening. As she progressed Jane found that her ease of playing and the quality of the note improved. An additional bonus was her increased enjoyment of playing.

Jane's example illustrates how the Technique can improve performance. So often skilled performers, be they in sport, music, acting, or whatever, have seemingly unimportant habits of body use that actually undermine their chances of success. It is not usually possible to correct such problems immediately; a course of basic lessons that deals with the person's whole body is needed first, then once the Technique has been mastered, it can be applied to improving a particular skill.

Mr G is a dentist, who came to me complaining of neck and shoulder pain. When we first met the muscles of his neck and shoulders were indeed tight, but so were those of his belly, back, arms and legs. We worked together to unravel what was cause and what was effect.

From this it became clear that the pains were caused by Mr G literally pulling himself out of shape in his work, mainly by an overcontraction of his chest and belly muscles and poking his head forwards. Once he realized he was doing this and was taught how to prevent it, the pains began to abate.

This kind of problem is common. For a variety of reasons people develop habits of body use which produce so much stress in the body that painful symptoms result. Finally it is important to notice that we did not attempt to treat the symptoms directly. Instead, we found the cause of the body misuse that underlay them.

Don't worry — this injection isn't for you..

MR G. IS A DENTIST — HE SUFFERED FROM NECK AND SHOULDER PAIN.....

Elizabeth K is a respected psychotherapist. Some of her colleagues had told her about the Alexander Technique and she decided that, although she had no specific problems, she would like to know how to use her body in a more natural way. When we began working together it was obvious that she was a very intelligent and sensitive person. She quickly felt the freedom and lightness in her body increasing. More interesting for her was the experience of the connection between thoughts, feelings, and the way the body works. She was already aware of the existence of this link from her own work with the emotions, but the closeness of the connection was a revelation to her. She was particularly fascinated by the direct link between thought, the aliveness of the body and positive emotional changes.

Elizabeth is an example of a growing number of people who take lessons in the Alexander Technique, not because of health or performance problems, but because they find it a valuable tool for improving their wellbeing and self-knowledge.

2.
WHY WE NEED ALEXANDER TECHNIQUE

BODY MISUSE AND MODERN LIVING

'We live in a time of rapid change' is a phrase in constant use these days. Usually, it is used to refer to technological advances, scientific breakthroughs and so on, but it also applies to us as a society – ideas change, different political parties come and go, social norms shift (note, for example, the recent upsurge in divorce). Obviously we as individuals are affected too. What do such upheavals do to our bodies, not to mention our minds and relationships? In simpler, more stable societies the body use of ordinary, healthy people is quite different from those we see in contemporary westerners. In the process of making his discovery Alexander began to think about the causes for this.

He suggested that under natural conditions only the creatures with good body use survive, those who are clumsy and slow perish. Under these relatively unchanging conditions successful creatures naturally tend to have good body use. But with the rise of agriculture and the growth of cities a great change occurred. The body was less and less used in a spontaneous and natural way. It was more and more restricted to a narrow range of activities. At the mental level, thought became ever more complex and the increase of formal education accentuated this.

In short there has been a rapid and increasing change in the demands on human beings which has caused a general change in the way humans operate. They have become less and less physical, more and more mental, more and more static, and more and more complicated. It has led one critic of civilization to call modern humans 'homo-sedens' – the 'sitting human'.

It must be remembered that human evolution has taken at least five million years, only the last 10,000 of which can be said to have been civilized. This would imply that our biology is 99.9 per cent based on the relatively unchanging demands of nature. Only a very small percentage has had time to adapt to the new and rapidly changing conditions of civilization.

Before modern time, the slow rate of change allowed humans to gradually and unconsciously adapt the body to new conditions. Now, however, it is we who change the environment, and we do it more and more rapidly. Think for a moment of your day, from when you wake up in the morning, and contrast it with what living in the wild must have been like: sleeping in a soft bed; being woken up by a sudden mechanical or electronic noise; the almost instantaneous change from dark to light as we switch on the bedside light in winter; sitting, in a chair at breakfast, in a bus or train or car, at work, after work; walking down a street on a hard pavement, often within a few feet of fast moving and noisy vehicles, each of which can be bigger, faster and noisier than any animal; reacting to events we cannot hear or see directly via telephone, radio and TV. Is it any wonder many of us become over-tense and collapse in a heap at the end of such a day?

Proprioception

The changes mentioned above are only a few of those that occur constantly in our everyday lives. In total they are more dramatic and wide ranging than we imagine. As a result of this tension in our bodies, the information our brains receive about where parts of the body are and what they are doing relative to each other, whether they are moving or still, is less reliable than when we lived in the wild. This information concerning the state of the body is called proprioception, and comes mainly from the joints, tendons and muscles. The importance of proprioception can hardly be exaggerated. It is the basis for balance, posture and movement. Even more fundamental, it is the basis for our sense of self. This aspect of proprioception is vividly illustrated by the neurologist Oliver Sacks, who reported one of his case studies about a woman who lost almost all proprioception. Her accompanying loss of her sense of self and her emotional, as well as physical, difficulties make harrowing reading.

Re-educating our proprioception

What we have not done, Alexander suggests, is to apply our reasoning to how we can learn to react in a better way to these changed circumstances and re-educate our proprioception so that it becomes reliable once more. We have not noticed the general deterioration in the way we use our bodies due to our loss of proprioceptive acuity. We do not consider the possible effect of the general misuse of our bodies on our ability to carry out both every-day and skilled actions, on our health and even on our underlying psychological state. Instead we only notice specific symptoms and then try to treat them in isolation. We do not see, for example, that our headache is connected to the way we are using our whole body.

Alexander was not suggesting that all our problems are caused by misuse of the body, but that it can be a factor which in many instances is the dominant one.

Moreover, almost all of us misuse our bodies to some extent, which has to affect us adversely in a variety of ways.

Diana K is a dancer. After a successful professional career, she began to question her work. This led her to explore various styles of dance and other disciplines including the Alexander Technique. In the course of her lessons she found that she was holding her body in a rather fixed and rigid way, especially when she began to dance. Although she was very flexible, the amount of movement she could coax from her body actually came from forcing it to move, and, as with many other dancers, this had led to nagging injury problems. As we worked she found that she could approach her dance in a more relaxed, natural way, opening up new creative opportunities for her dance and incidentally reducing her injury problems.

HOW MISUSE MANIFESTS ITSELF

When a number of scientists looked closely at the way most people stand, they came up with surprisingly similar results, results which did, in fact, differ quite markedly from the pictures we see in anatomy textbooks (see diagram A on page 38).

In most people the head and the pelvis are in front of the body (see diagram B on page 39). The curves of the neck and upper back are exaggerated and there is a flattening of the curve in the lower spine. Notice how the balance of the body is in front of the ankle joints.

In dancers we often see a different pattern (see diagram C on page 39). Here the neck and upper back are over straight and the lower back has a large curve, with the legs being stiff and straight. In such cases the balance of the body is further back, but the body is rather tense.

With students of the Alexander Technique the body tends to look more like that in diagram A, but in a free and natural way and with great individual variations. It must be emphasized that these changes, and others detailed later, are not the result of simply trying to stand up straight. They come about naturally when the body is allowed to use the proper mechanisms.

HOW ALEXANDER STOPPED MISUSING HIS BODY

The short answer to this question is by stopping pulling his head back and down and making himself shorter and narrower. Although this is factually correct, it does not tell us *how* he did it. And without the practical experience it is difficult to explain.

However the discoveries Alexander made can be described fairly simply. Studies have shown how we pull ourselves out of shape. The curves in the spine, for instance, are usually distorted, the ribs narrowed and the balance of the head disturbed, usually as the result of muscles contracting and shortening too much.

'Primary control'

The first step to preventing distortion of the spinal curves happening, Alexander discovered, was to refuse to act immediately. The next step was to achieve lengthening of the muscles by 'directing the head forward and up without stiffening and narrowing the back'. Alexander called this skill 'the primary control', primary because it is the first action that must be working correctly if proprioception and other senses are to be improved. This in turn allows improvements in balance, posture and movement – three key factors affecting health and performance. Refusing to act too hastily allows muscles to decontract, while operating the primary control allows muscles to lengthen by the mechanisms described below.

As we shall see later there is good reason to believe that the improvement in balance reduces muscle tension and the chance of damage to muscles and bones. Improved

(A)

Idealised posture.
(as shown in
anatomy textbooks).

WAYS OF STANDING.

B

'Normal' Posture.

C

Consciously trying to stand up straight.

posture is a part of this. The increases in the length and width of the trunk found as a result of taking lessons in the Alexander Technique may be important in reducing harmful pressures on the heart, lungs, stomach, intestines and other internal organs. This may explain some of the health improvements noted by Barlow and Tinbergen.

A LITTLE ANATOMY

To help in the understanding of these ideas, let us take a very simple look at the structure of the body. The head balances very freely on top of the spine at what is called the atlanto-occipital joint. This simply means the joint between the top vertebra (called the atlas-vertebra) and the bottom part of the skull which is called the occipital bone (vertebra is the name given to the bones that make up the spine).

The spine is made up of 33 (in most people) vertebrae, linked together by joints that allow different kinds and amounts of movement between them, depending on the part of the spine and its job. However, although there is movement between most individual bones, if we take the spine as a whole, it can be regarded as a long springy curved column. Like the springs of a car's suspension it holds the body up but compresses when we put weight on it – just as when people get into a car you can see the car go down a little bit – and if you really load the car up it gets lower still. This is a result of the springs bending.

'Lengthening'

If you look again at the diagrams on pages 38–39 you can see that the shape of the spine is different in the different diagrams. Bringing ourselves back into balance – by stopping the muscles from imposing the wrong forces – tends to bring the spine back into shape. Also, by taking the excessive forces off the spine, just like the car springs, it gets longer and so do its associated muscles.

atlanto-
occipital
joint .

THE HEAD AND NECK VERTEBRAE

The lengthening of a muscle and improvements in proprioception go together because the sensory parts of a muscle need a degree of stretch to function. Also from a mechanical point of view, a muscle is more powerful when it is lengthening than when it is shortening. This explains what Alexander meant by 'lengthening', what about 'widening'?

'Widening'
The ribs grow out from the upper part of the back from what are called the thoracic vertebrae. In the baby, whilst it is in the womb, the ribs grow to enclose the heart, lungs, stomach, and other organs. Muscles connect the ribs to each other, and to the pelvis, spine, shoulders and arms. These muscles, together with the diaphragm, control the movement of the ribs. If there is a wrong pattern of tension in any of the muscles, the ribs can be stiffened and held in too narrow or too wide a position. In most people they are held too narrow. This is due to the arm, chest and abdominal muscles in particular being too short and too tight in most of us.

The Alexander Technique releases these muscle patterns so that the curved ribs can widen out as a consequence of their natural springyness. Notice that the ribs are not widened by using muscular force, but simply are not held 'narrow' and so they can move more freely and without effortful breathing. This freer, more natural breathing pattern is often the first sign of change as a result of Alexander lessons. It is frequently accompanied by sigh of relief and a surprised, but happy smile with the question, 'That's so nice – how did it happen?' Often the release occurs, not when the teacher is working on the abdomen or chest as one might expect, but when their hands are on the neck. From very early on Alexander found that the neck was the key part of the primary control. He was not an anatomist and did not concern himself with being more precise than just talking about the neck. Later, when physicians and scientists first tried to understand why the Alexander

vertebra

disc

joint to pelvis

THE CURVES OF THE SPINE

HEAD RETRACTION
IN SITTING DOWN

BETTER BODY USE IN
SITTING DOWN

Technique was effective in a more exact way, they were tempted to look for particular parts of the neck – some voted for the muscles just outside the atlanto-occipital joint, others for the joints in the neck.

Alexander himself, however, did not speculate about which parts of the neck were important, but focused on the practical point that when the neck is stiff and short it pulls the head down, causing in some way, a shortening and narrowing of the body. Conversely, when the neck is allowed to release, and the head is directed forward and up, the trunk as a whole can be directed to lengthen and widen.

3.
HOW ALEXANDER TECHNIQUE HELPS

Having seen the detrimental effects of poor posture and misuse of the body generally, the question now is how can we go about learning to stop interfering with the balance of the body?

To find some answers to this question we need to go back to Alexander's own experience for, as you may already have guessed, learning the Technique is not just a matter of knowing what should happen and making it happen. If you have any doubts about this, try demonstrating to an Alexander teacher what you think you have learned so far from this book.

THREE FUNDAMENTAL DISCOVERIES

In some ways you are roughly at the point where Alexander was when he had made his original discoveries. However, when he first tried to apply his findings to himself during his public recitations, he found he slipped back to his old habits almost immediately. So Alexander had to start again. By very careful observation

47

of exactly what he did, he was led to three further
fundamental discoveries.

'End gaining' and the 'means whereby'
First, that the habits he was dealing with were far more
deep-rooted and powerful than he had at first thought.
The most serious of these, he found, was the tendency
to try to act immediately. The best analogy for this is
walking across a busy road: if we just 'do it', we are liable
to be run over; instead we have to stand at the kerbside,
look and wait until there is no traffic and it is safe. This
is an action we have to learn consciously and by repetition
– no doubt you remember being taught your 'kerb drill'
as a child. In the end the routine is almost automatic
(we will return to the importance of the 'almost' later).
This habit of going directly for things Alexander called
'end gaining'. Its opposite, the process of waiting,
observing and working out what must and must not
happen so we can perform the action safely and well he
called attending to the 'means whereby'. (Incidentally
it was learning these concepts from Alexander that led
Aldous Huxley to write his book *Ends and Means*.)

'Faulty sensory appreciation'
His second important realization was that these habits
were not just habits of action, but that, like the habit
of running our fingers through our hair, there were habits
of feeling (proprioception) underlying the habitual
actions. It was the habitual, unnoticed feelings from his
body that he was relying on to do the action. So much
so that, if he did prevent his habitual stiffening and
tightening before an action, it felt quite wrong to him.
This shows just how fundamental proprioception is and
how central proprioceptive habits are to the way we use
our bodies.

It is quite common for students, when they have been
helped to release their body, to feel twisted or that they
are leaning backwards or forwards, when in fact they
are now straight and vertical for the first time. As you
can guess this sets up a vicious circle preventing change.

'ATTENDING TO THE MEANS WHEREBY..'

Alexander called this kind of problem with our feelings 'faulty sensory appreciation'.

'Inhibition'

Recognizing this problem led Alexander to the third discovery. This was that before he did something, he had to stop so he could work out what he needed to do in order to carry it out well. This discovery of the need to stop he called 'inhibition'.

This turned out to be an unfortunate choice of words. Alexander made his discoveries before Freud's writing had become popularized and translated into English, but from then on 'inhibition' has been popularly thought of as something to do with the artificial supression of emotions and behaviour. Alexander, however, used the word in its physiological sense, meaning a healthy and natural self-control of unwanted and inappropriate

49

reactions, without any sense of suppressing spontaneity.

It is possible to see this concept in action when children wait to cross the road. They will chat, sing and even dance, wave to each other and so on in a spontaneous way, while they wait for a suitable time to cross the road. What Alexander was definitely not talking about was a wooden, stiff or overly serious attitude. In fact the story is told that one morning on the first teacher training course he gave, the students arrived looking rather serious. Alexander is supposed to have told them, 'I can't teach you when you're like that; go away and cheer up!'

He also said, 'When you stop doing the wrong thing, the right thing does itself.' Alexander knew from his own experience, that if he could maintain the inhibition, that is stopping the old habits coming back, and use the primary control, then the body moved and worked freely and naturally without any of the usual effort.

'WHEN YOU STOP DOING THE WRONG THING, THE RIGHT THING DOES ITSELF'

TOWARDS A SOLUTION

When Alexander found a way of integrating these discoveries in practice, he had found the answer to his problems. By recognizing the strength of his habits and the inappropriateness of 'end gaining', he was forced to look carefully at what he was doing and consider the 'means whereby' he was going to gain his end. In this process he had to overcome his 'faulty sensory appreciation' of how his body should be. This he did by 'inhibiting' his initial 'end gaining' way of working and instead, by ensuring he kept his 'directions' for operating the primary control, caused the body to work more naturally.

Like the kerb drill learnt by children this process requires repetition and time. Trying to force things to happen or going too quickly simply excites fear reflexes which block the possibility of free, natural body use. Instead we have to give time for the conscious thoughts of the directions to be laid down in the nervous system. This in turn will affect the general muscle tone, and through this, posture and movement will both change.

It is not surprising that it took Alexander so long to make his discovery and perfect the Technique in practice. Even with this written information, the Technique is very difficult to carry out in practice. Nor should this be any other way — no one expects to learn how to drive a car, for example, or play a musical instrument from just reading a book.

THE TEACHER'S ROLE

The work of the Alexander teacher is, of course, to be able to explain the ideas of the Technique and help to diagnose the student's problems and then to find out how to deal with them. But beyond that, what is vital to the student's learning of the Technique is the skilful use of the teacher's hands to give the experience needed. This way of using the hands is achieved by a long period of

NOONE EXPECTS TO LEARN HOW TO DRIVE A CAR OR PLAY
A MUSICAL INSTRUMENT FROM JUST READING A BOOK

training in which the teacher becomes so fluent in the
Technique, that they are able to use and apply the steps
Alexander discovered reliably to themselves. The result
is that they have a quality of muscle tone in their body
that allows them to transmit the same possibilities to
the muscles of the student. As a result the student can
be helped, not only to observe themselves and understand
what is being attempted, but above all to *experience* what
changes can be achieved and the quality of body use
required to gain these.

ALEXANDER'S METHOD

Let us go back and look in more detail at the actual process
Alexander went through to make and integrate his last
three discoveries. After much experiment he found that
he had to fool his brain to prevent it telling the muscles
to get ready in its old habitual way. For example when

he got ready to recite, instead of 'just doing it', he found that he had to:

1. refuse to do it immediately (inhibit);
2. give the directions for the primary control in sequence;
3. keep giving the directions until he was confident that he could use them to do whatever he wanted to do (that is he was attending to the means whereby);
4. while still sending the directions, he stopped and reconsidered what he actually wanted to do. He then made a fresh decision to be equally open to either
   a. doing something completely different or,
   b. going on to do the action or,
   c. doing nothing at all.

In each case, when he made his new decision he continued repeating his directions, that is consciously wishing his neck to be free, his head to go forward and up and his torso to lengthen and widen. These directions provided the 'means whereby' his body would work with the maximum ease and effectiveness as they operated the primary control.

This may sound a difficult and complicated procedure but, with the expert help of a teacher this essential practical skill is made much easier. The teacher can, by means of his hands, enable the student to experience the primary control working, while at the same time learning how to give the corresponding directions. Because the teacher has a very acute sense of what is happening in the student's muscles from his hands, he is able to ensure that the student really does keep the primary control working well during the action. Should this be lost at any time, the teacher can stop the student and take him back to the point where he lost it, so the student can pinpoint his problems and learn how to overcome them.

This is a gentle, delicate process involving non-judgemental awareness on the part of both teacher and student, combined with great attention being paid to what is actually happening. This very accurate observation and clear diagnosis, together with positive and practical help in the solution of difficulties, is the hallmark of good teaching.

4.
THINKING ABOUT ALEXANDER TECHNIQUE

What exactly is the Alexander Technique? Why do I need it? How many lessons do I need? How long does each lesson last? How can I find an Alexander teacher? How do I know if they are properly trained? What do lessons cost? What should I wear? These are just a few of the many questions people ask when considering whether or not to consult an Alexander teacher and in this chapter I will attempt to answer them, and some of the others that crop up regularly so you can approach the Technique fully informed and confident.

What is the Technique?
Briefly, it is a practical method for finding out what habits of body use we have and how we can prevent those which we find to be harmful.

Why do I need it?
The instinctive body responses to danger are often triggered inappropriately by everyday events in our rushed, highly technological society. (Think, for example,

of the effect the noise of traffic has on you.) We become
stressed and tense, and as a result pull our bodies out
of shape. This pattern quickly becomes habitual,
undermining not only performance but also health. The
Alexander technique enables us to recognize such
patterns *and* prevent them, allowing us to improve our
overall functioning and general level of wellbeing.

What are the basic ideas?

Use: How we use our body affects how it can function.
For example, trying to use a chisel as a screwdriver is
a *misuse* of it, causing it damage and preventing it being
used for its proper function of chiseling. Conversely using
the chisel as it should be used and keeping it sharp will
maintain its usefulness. Similarly our body will only work
at its best if we learn how to use it correctly.

Inhibition: The process of stopping the misuse of the body
is called inhibition. This involves a conscious refusal to
act in the old way so that a new and better way of using
the body can be found.

Sensory appreciation: To use the body well we have to
ensure that it is accurately informed of what it is doing.
Much of this information comes from proprioception. Due
to bad habits of body use this sensory appreciation is
faulty in most of us. With training it can be made more
reliable.

Primary control: To improve our sensory appreciation
we have to improve the way we use our body by learning
how to activate the primary control. This is done by
ensuring that the head, neck and trunk maintain a
dynamic relationship to maximize length and width in
the torso. Although this is difficult to explain in words
it can be quickly and effectively demonstrated by a
teacher.

Directions: For Alexander the body was always being
directed, consciously or subconsciously, well or badly, in

a new way or habitually, to prevent something or cause it. In the Technique we are concerned, firstly to prevent misuse due to subconsious, habitual directions and then build up the primary control with consciously chosen directions, leading to a better use of the body.

End gaining: Going directly for what we want, acting immediately, without thinking of what we are doing in the process, is what Alexander meant by this term. He recognized it as a central problem in learning of all kinds, especially the Technique.

Attending to the means whereby: This is the key to stopping the over hasty reactions caused by end gaining, which are often the cause of misuse. Inhibition is needed to stop the end gaining reactions. New directions are then given to build up the means whereby the end can best be gained, step by step. In practice this usually means giving the directions that will build up the primary control.

How many lessons do I need?
Alexander prescribed a minimum course of 30 lessons. Some teachers suggest 20. The number you need will depend on what you want to achieve and what problems you have. Mr G's symptoms improved in a matter of six lessons, although it took longer for him to learn the new use that prevented them from returning. For Diana K, on the other hand, the lessons were not undertaken to deal with any specific problems, and she took lessons intermittently over three years, using them to re-form her dance.

How long does each lesson last?
Alexander found that 30 minutes was the time he needed to make useful changes. Less experienced teachers may take about 40 minutes. For most students this is the maximum time they can maintain the level of attention required and benefit from the changes which are occurring.

How can I find an Alexander teacher?

As advertising by teachers is restricted by their professional body you are unlikely to find lurid advertisements for them in newspapers and magazines. They may list themselves in the telephone directory under the Alexander Technique. The sure way of finding a teacher is to write to the secretary of The Society of Teachers of the Alexander Technique (STAT) whose address is at the back of the book (see p. 99) and they will send you a complete list of qualified teachers.

How do I know if a teacher is properly qualified?

A teacher should have a certificate issued by The Society of Teachers of the Alexander Technique (STAT), or by F M Alexander himself, or by The American Center for the Alexander Technique, or by one of the national societies of teachers now being set up in several countries. All these societies are affiliated to STAT and so a certificate from one of these societies should say this on it. If you are in any doubt contact the secretary of STAT.

What do lessons cost?

The price of a lesson will vary depending on the experience of the teacher and their overheads. For example a practice in central London is much more expensive to maintain than one in the country. Fees range from about £5 to £15 in Britain, $20 to $60 in the USA and DM30 to DM60 in Germany, for example. There is no necessary connection between the quality of a lesson and the fee charged. If you can, I suggest you try two or three teachers before deciding who you want to work with and how much you want to pay.

What should I wear?

Ordinary, everyday clothes that are easy to move in are the best. Very tight jeans or very high heels are not recommended unless these are what you normally wear. I say this because the Alexander Technique is about how

4. THINKING ABOUT ALEXANDER TECHNIQUE

to live your *normal* life in a better way; it is not something
that requires special exercises or clothing. You do not
need to take your clothes off for a lesson.

Do I have to avoid eating and drinking before a lesson?
Only in as far as a heavy meal or too much alcohol can
make you drowsy and less able to attend to the lesson.

Can I ask questions?
Yes!

What should I ask?
It is a good idea to clear up any basic queries before the
first lesson, such as what are the teacher's experience,
qualifications and fees. Also find out whether they think
they can help you with your particular needs, and how
often you should have lessons and how many. Ask what
happens if you cannot do as many as they suggest. Find
out if they are able to take you on now, or if they have
a long waiting list. If they do, ask if they can recommend
other teachers.

What should I tell the teacher?
It is a good idea to be as clear as you can about why you
want lessons. What do you want to achieve? How much
time will you have? If you have any particular medical
problems be sure to mention them. Teachers will not wish
to pry into your private life but, if you think anything
of a personal nature is causing difficulties, it might be
worth mentioning.

   Additionally, if you read through the next sections and
think you may have problems with the sort of things that
happen in a lesson you should warn the teacher.

What will I be asked by the teacher?
Teachers usually like to have your home and work
telephone numbers so that they can contact you if any
changes of appointment are needed. If you are receiving

Life-enhancement... OK... Fine. anything more specific?

IT IS A GOOD IDEA TO BE AS CLEAR AS YOU CAN ABOUT WHY YOU WANT THE LESSONS.

medical treatment they may ask you to check that your doctor approves of you taking lessons. If you have not discussed it already, the teacher will probably ask you why you want lessons and if you have any particular problems.

What happens in the first few lessons?
Exactly what happens depends of course on you, the teacher and your particular needs. What follows is only a very approximate guide based on my own experience. At the first lesson I generally sit down with a student and go through the various questions I have just indicated. This usually takes five or ten minutes. When I feel we have go to know each other a little, I explain that I'd like to place my hands on the neck and shoulders as the student sits down, to feel what is going on. This gives me a rough idea of how tense the person is and gets us more used to each other. In particular it gives the student an experience of being touched in a non-invasive and non-judgemental way.

60

PUTTING MY HANDS ON THEIR NECK AND
SHOULDERS .... GIVES ME A ROUGH IDEA HOW
TENSE A PERSON IS ... .

With one hand remaining on the neck I ask the student to stand up in the normal way. Having done this, we swap places and I copy the student's movement pattern, so he or she can see and feel what it is like from the outside. I then briefly explain what I saw in the pattern and how it is affecting their body. From this I go on to give a very brief outline of Alexander's discoveries and to demonstrate the effect inhibition and direction have on me. The difference is usually clear cut so that we can swap back. By using my hands, I can bring about the changes needed in the way the student uses his or her body so that they can feel the difference in themselves. Usually, students quickly feel that they are taller, lighter and move more easily.

As soon as it is possible, I ask students to start to think of the directions, so they can learn to use the primary control for themselves. In the early lessons this can only happen when my hands make the necessary change for them, but with time most students learn how to use it for themselves.

The early lessons are confined to very simple situations, like sitting, standing and lying down. We concentrate on these because they are simple, everyday actions. The aim is to help in learning how to apply the Technique to any action. As the lessons progress, more complicated examples can be dealt with.

5.
STAGES OF
LEARNING

Each individual will vary in the rate they learn the Technique. Much depends on how much misuse their bodies have already received and how severe their problems are before the lessons start. Consequently, the following outline of stages is by no means definitive, although it does provide a general guide to the stages of progress experienced by students of the Technique.

FIRST STAGE

The first stage in learning the Technique is being able to experience the activating of the primary control through the teacher's use of her hands. In some students this is immediate – they can feel the changes in their musculature together with the lengthening and widening of their trunk. They feel lighter and freer when they move. Some will also report psychological experiences.

The majority of students are a little slower in reaching the first stage. In my own case, although the early lessons were pleasant, I did not feel any specific or clear changes for about six months. However, most students do feel changes before then. In a few cases the student will not feel any changes at all. A senior colleague of mine tells of a man he was teaching, who had received 30 lessons and obviously did not feel anything. My colleague asked him why he was continuing to take lessons. 'Well', said the man, 'I've had to buy new jackets because I'm too broad for my old ones, I've also had to buy new shoes as my feet have grown and my children tell me that I'm a much nicer man to live with.'

This cautionary tale is important. It illustrates graphically the fact that the Technique is actually concerned with making objective improvements in the way we use our bodies, and that these objective changes may not be accompanied by any subjective changes. Alternatively, the changes experienced may not correspond to the objective changes. This is illustrated by a student who, when he was asked to free his neck, actually stiffened it. With another student, when I asked her to let her head go forward and up, she actually pulled it back.

These cases illustrate how our habits are deeply rooted in our ideas, our way of living and, in particular, in our way of responding to a demand being placed on us. Rather like animals when they sense something unusual, we automatically stiffen in response to a demand whereas, what is actually required in a non-survival situation, is that we remain quiet but alert for anything of interest. This allows us to respond in a free and effortless way. To help the students just mentioned, the trick was to ask them to think of stiffening and pulling the head back. This produced the respective freeing of the neck and releasing forward of the head! A further warning to be taken from these examples is the power of words. Each individual has his or her own personal set of associations for a particular word. This is especially true with habits.

RATHER LIKE ANIMALS WHEN THEY SENSE SOMETHING UNUSUAL, WE STIFFEN..

SECOND STAGE

As the lessons proceed, and the objective changes are repeated with the help of the teacher, the student enters the second stage. In this stage the student begins to be able to give the directions for herself when she is still and the teacher's hands are on her. With some students this is a quick and simple matter. They are tuned in to their bodies and can, as Alexander phrased it 'ask nicely' for the greater freedom in their body use. However, for most of us, it is at this stage we meet the problem of habit. Take Peter F for example. He is a rock musician, whose work requires a lot of travelling, very hard and loud playing, and irregular hours. In his own words he is a 'go-getter'. His body is strong and in Alexander terms rather stiff and hard, a stance his body use reflected. His movements were very quick and rather angular, he was constantly ready to go. When we began working, I quickly realized that the problem we had to deal with was getting Peter to stop. Until he could be persuaded to stop, mentally as well as physically, he would be unable to

65

experience the Technique, let alone apply it for
himself.

Peter began to see what was needed but was unable
to do anything about it. How could he? The only way he
knew of making something happen was to make it
happen! The idea of letting something happen by not
doing something else was not only impossible for him
in practice but inconceivable in theory. The way through
for us was to let him feel me as I acted in the way he
did and to compare that with when I stopped and gave
my directions. Then, while he was thinking about this,
I would guide him through the action.

As he was busy, there were gaps in his lessons and often
we had to go back to the beginning. As Peter learned to
stop and just leave his body alone, he began to experience
the working of the primary control. Gradually, he was
able to learn how to give his directions without trying
to make something specific happen. Otherwise this
usually resulted in either stiffening, or, if he tried to relax,
a collapse of one part of the body, which makes it stiffen
somewhere else. This led him to the third stage of being
able to continue to give his directions when I guided him
as he moved, for example, from sitting to standing.

THIRD STAGE

This third stage is similar to the stage Alexander reached
when he found he could both give his directions and recite.
The difference is that with the help of the teacher, the
students are corrected almost automatically and as they
go into action. This means that quite often, we do not
have to explicitly teach the method Alexander used on
himself to fool his habits at the critical moment of starting
an action.

When students reached this stage with Alexander, he
worked with them on two particular procedures. First,
he concentrated on the process of bending forward, either
when sitting or standing and putting the hands on the
back of a chair. These he called the positions of

mechanical advantage or more familiarly 'monkey'.
Through working on this procedure systematically, a
student can learn how to do something with their hands,
be it writing, drawing, washing the dishes, adjusting the
controls of a car or playing a musical instrument, whilst
maintaining the primary control.

The second procedure was that of using the voice and
breathing to produce a particular sound, called 'the
whispered ah'. This leads to being more skilful in
anything that involves the voice or breathing, in giving
lectures, singing, talking on the phone or playing a wind
instrument, for example.

Between them, these two procedures provide useful
prototypes for studying the whole range of human actions,
from walking and running to dancing, cycling, jumping,
lifting, carrying, practising yoga, tai chi, or martial arts,
making expressive movements and to the study of body
language. Each of these deserves a book to itself but their
practice must be learnt from a teacher.

FOURTH STAGE

The fourth stage is one in which the student is able to
maintain the primary control without guidance in an
increasing number of activities and situations. At first,
it may only be possible in a reliable way in the teaching
room and only then for simple activities. As you gain in
experience this can extend outside to more and more
activities.

An example may help. Betty G is a secretary, an
amenable, efficient and helpful person. Her boss was used
to her being obliging and tended to ask her to work
overtime. Sometimes she resented this but she didn't
know how to say no. Her boss was rather overbearing
and she was rather timid. If she argued with her boss,
the boss always won.

One evening, when she was due to have an Alexander
lesson, her boss asked her to work overtime again. This
time, rather than saying yes or arguing, she gave her

IF SHE ARGUED WITH HER BOSS, THE BOSS ALWAYS WON.

directions, then, firmly but politely said, 'No, I have an important appointment.' The boss was so surprised by her straightforward polite refusal that she (the boss) had nothing to argue about and so had to agree. This saying no to old patterns by pausing and giving the new directions is equally effective in less emotional situations.

FAILURES

As with many areas of human endeavour, Alexander lessons sometimes do not work. This may be only a temporary hitch, we all have occasional difficulties in learning anything. Sometimes, however, it may be a more long term problem.

The most common problem is that of attitude. Occasionally, people who are sent to have lessons by well-meaning relatives or friends, are simply not interested. In other cases, the person is looking for a specific, quick and easy cure for their problem. They expect a teacher

68

to sort them out with a maximum of speed and a minimum of interference with their normal life. In Alexander terms these people are 'end-gainers' who find this sometimes slow and painstaking work frustrating. They haven't got time for bothering about such things, they say.

Another problem of attitude, is sometimes found in people who are practising one of the various growth methods now popular. Before I go on, let me make it clear that I am in no way criticizing any of these methods but simply the fixed attitudes some people have towards a particular method. Some examples may illustrate these problems. Brenda A is a teacher who has suffered from neck and shoulder pains for some years. She took a form of posture training which taught her how to stand and sit correctly. Although the ideas themselves were sensible, they failed to deal with the habits underlying Brenda's neck and shoulder problems. When we came to work with each other, I found that as she got ready either to stand or sit, she would put one foot backwards first. This caused her whole body to stiffen and become noticeably shorter. We discussed the problem. I explained what I saw and felt in her body and demonstrated it. However, because it was such a part of her, Brenda did not feel it at first. The habit, especially because she had learned that it was the only way to move, was so powerful that no other possibility could even be considered. She could not allow herself the possibility of acting in a different way, not because she was resisting my work but because her feelings told her anything else was impossible. Gradually, as we continued our work, and I made it clear that I was not attacking the method she had learned but her response to it, she was able to take a fresh look at herself, and gradually learn how to let her body be free and light when she moved.

Robert J is a busy public relations officer for a large company. His work involves many meetings and planning conferences. He had developed an interest in psychology and various forms of psychotherapy, and through these he had made contact with some of the emotional factors in his life. He came to me for lessons as he was curious about the Alexander Technique. It was quickly apparent that Robert was over-relaxed, that is his body was very heavy and unresponsive. When I talked to him about this, he explained that he was feeling what was happening in his body and various emotions coming from our work together.

I explained that the focus of our work was attending in a more general way to what we wanted to do and what we were doing to ourselves in the process. As a part of that, feelings and emotions were important. However, if we concentrated purely on the feelings and emotions, we made it impossible to produce the improvements in the way we use our body and mind that, in turn, would have positive effects on our feelings and emotions. More generally, feelings and emotions tell us about what has happened or what we imagine might happen. They do not tell us what we can decide on or how we can achieve it. What we want is not to work against our feelings or emotions, but to have a clear perception of what is good for us.

Part of deciding is based on emotions: 'I want to do something'. The wanting provides the motive power. The how, the shaping of the wish, seeing how it fits in with a broader perspective, requires conscious thought. This is the aspect we are dealing with in the Technique. Robert agreed with this and I was able to demonstrate to him that his body could be lighter and freer with this new way of thought. However, this was not Robert's interest. He wanted to continue his exploration of feelings and emotions in his way, because this was what felt better and more important to him. This was his prerogative. The Technique is not concerned with conditioning or hypnosis or other methods of influencing people without their free will. It is concerned with the use of observation and choice and people must be free to exercise these facilities.

One reason students give for stopping lessons is money, or rather the lack of it. I would suggest, that if this is

IT WAS QUICKLY APPARENT THAT ROBERT WAS
OVERRELAXED AND HIS BODY HEAVY AND
UNRESPONSIVE.

THE REASON STUDENTS GIVE FOR STOPPING LESSONS IS LACK OF MONEY.

the reason for anyone stopping, they should talk to their teacher. I know of no Alexander teacher who would refuse tuition through a student's inability to pay full fees.

Sometimes a teacher fails to 'speak the student's language'. It is difficult frankly to relate well to everyone and this is one of the reasons why I suggested trying two or three different teachers before you decide with which one you want to study.

WHY IT TAKES A LONG TIME TO LEARN

As you can see from the examples given so far, there are real problems to overcome in learning the Technique. Psychological and physical restrictions are so intertwined as to be inseparable. This is why Alexander talked about the 'self' rather than mind or body. Such problems cannot be solved quickly, they are part of ourselves. Instead we have to allow growth and development to work. This

72

allows us to integrate the psychological and physical changes brought about by the Technique at our own pace.

WHY INDIVIDUAL LESSONS ARE NECESSARY

Each of us is a unique human being with individual requirements. Above all, each of us has to receive the necessary stimulus to learn how to use our own primary control. We can learn a lot from groups, most of the material given in this book can be taught that way. However, the essential experience of the primary control actually working in our bodies requires the physical intervention of a teacher. This is rather like tuning a musical instrument or a car engine; each individual instrument or engine has to be physically adjusted for it to work well. The very complexity of our body-mind makes this a demanding and delicate task. This is one of the reasons for the long training of teachers and the need for the sensitivity in the use of their hands. The process of adjustment is intensely personal, it needs time and a supportive, unstressed situation. Further, much of what is exchanged between student and teacher is private. The confidence needed to allow the fundamental changes required by the Technique often needs the confidentiality of private lessons.

There is a place for group work in the Technique. With my students I like to have monthly group meetings where we can discuss the Technique, new information can be given, and some practical work done. However, this requires continuing individual work to ensure each person can take on board whatever practical changes are suitable for them.

WHY 'HOW TO DO IT' BOOKS DO NOT WORK

Books, like groups, can inform, enthuse, and influence. 'How to do it' books, however, do not show *you* how to do it. Your particular needs and difficulties cannot be dealt with and it is precisely with these areas that the Technique is concerned.

6.
SCIENCE AND THE ALEXANDER TECHNIQUE

EARLY SCIENTIFIC SUPPORT

Some years after he arrived in England, Alexander had dinner with Sir Charles Sherrington, the greatest physiologist of modern times. Sherrington made some of the most significant discoveries on the way nerves control muscles and how the muscles are vital in informing the nervous system of what it should and should not do next. At a personal level the meeting was not a success. However, Sherrington supported Alexander's work for the rest of his life. He did this because he knew from his laboratory studies, and those of his colleague, Rudolf Magnus, that the neck and the head play a crucial role in the control of posture, balance and movement.

As he said, 'Mr Alexander has done a service to the subject [the physiology of posture and movement] by insistingly treating each act as involving the whole integrated individual, the whole psycho-physical man.

To take a step is an affair, not of this or that limb solely,
but of the total neuro-muscular activity of the moment
– not least of the head and neck.'

With the publication of Magnus' work in the 1920s,
detailing the roles of the head and neck, physiologists
and doctors who recognized Alexander's work began to
speculate about the mechanisms of the Technique – how
the body produced the changes we observe. Meanwhile,
the number of physicians and surgeons seeing the benefit
of the Technique increased to the point where 19 of them
wrote a letter to the *British Medical Journal*, urging that
the Alexander Technique be included in medical
training.

EXPERIMENTAL EVIDENCE

The evidence lacking in all this was that of direct
scientific experiment, although this requires much time
and money. At the end of the Second World War, however,
experimental studies did begin in Britain and the
USA.

Doctor Barlow
In Britain, Doctor Wilfred Barlow, while in the army
medical service, had begun to study young army recruits.
These first experiments by Barlow were simple: a tape
measure was hung from the back of the head; the length
of tape between the back of the head and the bottom of
the neck was measured, first when the person was
standing and then when they sat down. During the
process of sitting there was a shortening of the distance
between these points due to the head being pulled back.
The minimum distance was measured twice for each of
56 cadets and the average taken. All showed some
shortening. Out of the total number of cadets, 45 had a
shortening of over 1 inch and only 3 were aware they
had shortened. Even when the cadets were asked to focus
on the shortening, only 12 could feel it. When asked to
stop the shortening from happening, only 7 were able

to do so. 39 still had shortening of over 1 inch even though they thought that they had not shortened. This clearly demonstrates Alexander's point about the inaccuracy of our feelings, and the fact that we cannot make something happen just by trying when our feelings are so inaccurate.

FEELINGS CAN BE INACCURATE — SOME THOUGHT THEIR NECK HAD NOT SHORTENED WHEN IT HAD..

By asking subjects to stand in a standard position using a method developed by Professor J M Tanner, Barlow photographed a person from the front, side and back. He was able to analyse their posture from these photographs and reliably score the quality of their posture.

Barlow gave lessons to a group of 40 students from the Royal College of Music in London. They were photographed in the standard position before and after the course of lessons. Before the course the men had an average of 11 faults and at the end only 5. For the women the average faults were reduced from 9 to 4. These results were compared with a group of 44 students from the Central School of Speech and Drama in London who did not receive Alexander lessons. They were, however, given exercises aimed at improving posture. In this group the men deteriorated slightly from an average of 10.6 faults to 11.7. The women also deteriorated from 7.5 to 7.9.

As a comparison to these two groups, Barlow went on to measure 112 female physical education teacher students. The average number of defects in this group was 8.5. This suggests that even fit young people in our society have postural problems.

Only the students from the Royal College of Music showed an increase in height and shoulder width. All the results were assessed independently by Professor Tanner. In addition the teachers at the Royal College of Music made the following points in their report on the students' progress:

1. All the students improved physically in terms of their singing and acting abilities.
2. The students were easier to teach and had become more psychologically balanced.
3. The rate of improvement varied greatly between students.
4. The success of the students in an important singing competition was far greater than could have been expected.

ONLY ROYAL COLLEGE OF MUSIC STUDENTS
SHOWED AN INCREASE IN HEIGHT AND
SHOULDER WIDTH...

5. In their opinion the Alexander Technique was the best method they had experienced for helping a singer's performance and should form the basis of a singer's training.

Doctor Barlow's work clearly shows the effect of the Technique on posture and on the level of performance. Evidence for health improvements came from his clinical experience as a consultant in physical medicine at a London hospital.

Professor Jones

Professor F P Jones, working at Tufts University near Boston in the USA, used a different approach. He preferred to measure muscle activity and movement patterns for unguided and guided movements. Straightening up from a slumped sitting position is usually associated with a sense of effort. When the muscle activity is measured (called electromyographs or EMG's), there is more activity in the main neck muscles. However, when an Alexander teacher prevents the usual habitual stiffenings, the movement feels easier and the EMG records show less activity.

Using X-ray photographs, Jones was able to show that the Alexander movements resulted in an increase in the length of the sternomastoid muscles. These are key muscles in the control of head position and movement. You can feel them on either side of your throat and see them particularly clearly on dancers struggling to hold a position and on actresses trying to show strong emotions on TV soap operas. Another interesting find from the X-ray photographs was that there was an increase in the width of the discs between the neck vertebrae in Alexander subjects. Also, the X-rays showed a forward movement of the centre of gravity of the head. In other words an Alexander subject was taller, her neck was freer and the head had moved forward and up.

Jones used his techniques on the movement from sitting to standing. His movement photographs show a quicker and more direct movement. Unfortunately, he did not publish records of the muscle activity during the movement. Professor Finn Boyson-Møller of the University of Copenhagen and I therefore repeated the experiments using movement photographing equipment developed at the University of Copenhagen. In this experiment we also used a force platform. This is a piece of equipment which measures the size and direction of forces on it. Professor Jones had used one, but not in combination with the photographic and EMG measurements. Carrying out simultaneous recordings has the advantage of showing how these three measurements are related.

Our measurements showed that a guided movement required less force, used less muscle activity and was smoother and quicker than the habitual.

One problem with using photographic techniques is that slow movements are lost and taking measurements from the photograph leads to errors. For these reasons I went on to use a new electronic movement measurement system called Coda 3. The results of a pilot study allowed me to measure the speed and direction changes between someone moving in their habitual way, then trying to move faster and then using the Alexander Technique without guidance.

The results showed that using the Alexander Technique gave a more consistently upward movement with less wasted downward and backward movements of the body. As a result the movement took less time and force. In short it was more efficient.

Startle pattern

In other experiments Professor Jones studied the startle pattern. This is the typical reaction of someone when they are startled, for example, by a sudden unexpected noise. Jones found that the pattern always began in the neck and spread down the muscles of the body. It retracted the head, raised the shoulders, flattened the chest, straightened the arms and bent the legs. When one looks

retracted head

raised shoulders

flattened chest

straightened arms

bent legs

loss of bottle

STARTLE PATTERN

at people in the streets, it would seem that the startle pattern is more and more the norm for people as they get older. The balance of the head is changed, the neck is shorter and pulled forwards. The head is pulled backwards by the sternomastoid and trapezius muscles, just as these muscles tensed in the habitual movements shown earlier.

Sway analysis
What happens to our balance if we prevent this stiffening? A good measure of this is what is called sway analysis. When we stand, we do not stand still, we sway a little. Usually, this is not noticeable, but if we are drunk or have damage to some parts of the brain, the sway becomes exaggerated. Using a force platform we can analyse the sway, how much, how fast. Dr Roger Soames and I at the University of London plan to carry out experiments to establish the effects of Alexander lessons on sway shortly.

Moving the centre of balance

As you can see from the various drawings the result of Alexander lessons is usually a more upright standing position and it is evident that the body is more aligned. This was checked in detail by Dr David Garlick at the University of New South Wales in Australia. He found that Alexander lessons move the centre of balance of the body backwards, confirming Barlow's and my findings.

QUALITY OF PERFORMANCE

Doctor Barlow's study with students singing showed that there was a correlation between the objective posture changes and the reports on the students' performance from their professors. Jones was able to show that not only did a singer and others listening to her feel that the voice and breathing were improved, but there are measurable objectives changes in the sound as recorded by spectral analysis.

BLOOD PRESSURE

Both Jones and Barlow report cases of reductions in blood pressure in hypertensive students. To look more closely at this in normal subjects, Michael Nielsen of Aarhus University in Denmark and I carried out experiments on musicians under stress before and after Alexander lessons. These showed a significant drop in blood pressure.

BREATHING

Doctor Barlow found the Technique useful in dealing with breathing problems. Doctor Garlick and his team have investigated breathing and found that it is deeper and slower in people who have had Alexander lessons.

In the USA Dr John Austin measured both lung capacity and the maximum rate at which people could breathe out, the latter being a very good measure of how well the lungs are working. Both measures showed a significant improvement after a course of Alexander lessons.

DIGESTIVE PROBLEMS

Doctor Barlow found that the Technique helped with various disorders of the digestive system. No experimental studies have yet been published, but Barlow's clinical findings, and those of other doctors, confirm cases reported by Alexander. Alexander hypothesized that the problems helped by the Technique were caused by the high pressures from narrowing and pulling down, producing a downward movement of various internal organs. By restoring the length and width of the torso, the Technique makes possible the return of these organs to their normal positions and functioning.

Much work remains to be done to investigate the effects of the Technique more thoroughly. To this end the Alexander Research Trust has been set up and appeals for donations to fund further research. This is important for several reasons. Firstly, by documenting the benefits of the Technique, its usefulness will be more widely appreciated. Secondly, uncovering how the Technique achieves what it does will help us to understand it better. As a result we may find more effective ways of teaching it and contribute to a deeper understanding of the human being.

7.
HOW CAN I
HELP MYSELF?

Part of learning the Technique is finding out how to apply it to our own lives and interests. In this chapter I have sketched out some ideas about ways of doing this and I hope you will find them a useful addition to the practical work you do with a teacher. Throughout this chapter I am assuming that you are taking or have taken Alexander lessons. (This is in no way meant to be a 'how to' book.)

LYING WITH THE HEAD ON BOOKS

Most teachers will, as a part of at least some of their lessons, teach lying with the head on books. Please note, that this is not how we suggest you go to sleep. We use this procedure to give the maximum possibility for bringing the body into good shape. All that is needed is a warm room, a table covered with a blanket or a piece of carpeted floor and some paperback books. The principle of the exercise is, that by supporting the body on flat firm

LYING WITH THE HEAD ON BOOKS

surfaces, the muscles not only relax but the shape of the
body changes, allowing the spine to lengthen, the ribs
to widen and the head to rock forwards on the top of the
neck.

What height of books do I need?
The number of books needed depends on your height and
the size of your spinal curves. The easiest way of getting
a rough idea of how many books you need is to stand
normally with your bottom and shoulders against a wall,
then measure the distance between the back of your head
and the wall. If you add 1 inch to this distance that is
the approximate height of books you need. Your teacher
can give you more precise information.

How to lie down
As you will have found out in your lessons just doing
something always causes shortening. Instead you need
to pause and give your directions. It is useful to
experiment with different ways of lying down to avoid
building up rigid habitual ways of trying to do it right.
When you are lying down in the position shown in the
illustration above stop for a moment and instead of
trying to get comfortable, remember the problems of

86

blindly trusting your feelings. Rather just let your head rest on the books and your back rest on the table or the floor. Allow yourself to enjoy the experience. By this I do not mean pretend it is good if it is not. If you feel pain, please talk to your Alexander teacher and if necessary see a doctor. If you are not comfortable after you have stopped, then do move and repeat the stage.

Without losing your sense of enjoyment and your awareness of the back and head being supported, think of the neck being free as you have learned from your lessons. As the neck releases, the head, relative to the neck, is rocked forwards by the upthrust from the books. Just give permission for this to happen. The result of the neck releasing and the head going forwards is the lengthening of the spine and widening of the torso. In a lesson situation the teacher's hands bring this about. When you are on your own, it is your own giving of the directions that makes this possible. Of course, in a lesson the teacher's hands are used to help you give the directions but they are not a substitute for you giving them. Other directions that are useful are for releasing and lengthening the arms and legs (these will be taught by your teacher when you are ready). The important thing to remember here is not to concentrate on any particular part of the body. The primary control has to be kept operating while we extend our attention to include the limbs. Don't forget the primary control and only think of the limb you are working on.

SITTING

Sitting puts more stress on the spine than standing, so it is not surprising that people who sit a lot, particularly if they drive, are liable to back pain. How you sit can have a big effect on your chances of avoiding pain. Sitting slumped, particularly if you are leaning forwards, increases the pressure on the discs of the spine. Having lessons in the Technique will help reduce slumping considerably. Working with your teacher on the

particular demands of your work and interest can help
with these areas of your life.

If you have to sit for long periods, you may find the
concept of the pelvic support useful. This idea was
developed by John Gorman, an engineer, who suffered
from back pain. His reasoning is interesting, even though
it is not generally accepted as yet. When we sit in a
balanced way on a hard flat surface our pelvis and lower
spine are roughly in the position shown in diagram A
opposite. If, however, we are tired, we slump. This is
the typical position people come to if they sit unsupported
for any length of time (see diagram B, opposite).

Unfortunately designers and ergonomists have
mistaken this habitual posture, due to misuse and
fatigue, for the natural. Accordingly, they have designed
seats to fit this pattern. Although there have been some
improvements, at least in car seat design, in recent years,
most people sit as shown in diagram B opposite, even
in well-designed seats. This is because of the strength
of their earlier habits and the lack of support for the
pelvis. Diagram C opposite shows a typical example.
Compare this with diagram D on the same page, where
a pelvic support is used. The difference in the curve of
the lumbar spine is obvious, particularly at the bottom.

As most slipped discs are in the lower two joints of the
lumbar spine, it is tempting to suggest that correcting
the lumbar curve will prevent such damage in the spine.
For more active sitting it is often better to do away with
the back rest. Using a firm chair which can tilt forwards
about 10 to 15 degrees, helps in stabilizing the pelvis.
Raising the seat height so that the angle between the
trunk and the thighs is about 120 degrees helps
further.

What needs to be stressed is that it is important not
to force yourself to sit up straight. A famous French horn
player found this to his cost. Knowing from experience
the importance of good posture for playing his instrument,
he had always prided himself on sitting up straight.
Unfortunately, this was actually sitting up stiff and the

BALANCED SITTING.

SLUMPING

TYPICAL 'NORMAL' SITTING
IN A CHAIR OR CAR SEAT

SITTING WITH A PELVIC
SUPPORT.

result was two slipped discs. Forced to reconsider, he took Alexander lessons and found how to sit freely. Also, he saw that his back problem was a part of general pattern of stiffening and that another part of this general pattern of stiffening was bad breathing. As a result, his playing improved as well as his back.

The kind of chairs I have talked about are aids to sitting in an easy upright way. They are not a substitute for it – you can slump or strain in the best designed chairs. Through using the Technique you will be able to make the best of the good chairs and cope better with the bad ones you are bound to meet.

SITTING ON THE FLOOR

With the popularity of yoga and meditation many adults like to sit on the floor, as do many children. Such sitting is natural and has advantages over bad chairs. However, it is important to remember that habit is at work in all situations. Sitting on the floor does not stop bad habits of body use. Too often we see people slumped or strained when sitting on the floor, often they try to prop themselves up with cushions. A simple help is to sit on a pile of telephone directories. The number of books needed can be judged by the rule that when sitting cross-legged, the knees should not be higher than the hip joints. Please note, if you are very stiff, this is not true and I advise you to consult your Alexander teacher.

EXERCISE

Doing sport or exercises comes from the natural urge to move. Animals in the wild do not need them, neither do so-called primitive peoples. This is not surprising, as moving quickly and well is essential for survival in nature. As humans have become civilized, they use their bodies less and less. Thus there is an argument for doing exercises to give the body a chance to 'work out'. The problem is that not only have we underused our bodies,

I don't suppose you also make
a robot that presses
        the buttons ?. . . .

AS HUMANS HAVE BECOME MORE CIVILISED THEY HAVE
USED THEIR BODIES LESS.

but we have also learned to misuse them. If we don't deal
with the misuse and eliminate it, we will exercise the
misuse along with our body. It is like trying to drive a
badly maintained car, something is going to go wrong.
You have to stop and mend the defects as a first step.

For athletes who have used the Technique the result
has been an improvement in their performance and a
reduction in injuries. Take Paul Collins, an international
level marathon runner, who represented his country at
the 1952 Olympic Games. Knee injuries forced him to
stop running for many years. Later, he came across the
Alexander Technique and after having lessons, he noticed
that his knees were better. He began running again and
now at the age of 60 holds world records in running for
veterans.

91

Howard Paine was an Olympic level hammer thrower.
At the age of 40 he thought he was 'over the hill'. He,
too, came across the Alexander Technique. The result
was a marked increase in the length of his throw and a
greater enjoyment of his sport.

At a more mundane level a number of colleagues and
I took running lessons from Paul Collins. In these he
showed us how to apply the Technique to running. The
effect was electrifying: the usual sense of effort and slog
vanished, running became a joyful expression of our
bodies' natural abilities, rather than something we
imposed on them by willpower. At an objective level we
could see the kind of movement change from that of the
normal runner you see everyday in the street forcing
themselves along, to the style of Steve Cram and other
top level runners.

Exercise does not have to be strenuous to do you good.
Recent research shows we do best with the equivalent
of walking for one hour a day. Elaine T is a research
chemist whose boyfriend likes fell walking. He is tall and
long-legged whereas Elaine is short and plump. When
they first met, she naturally wanted to share his interest,
but found she could not keep up with him. For quite
different reasons she began taking Alexander lessons and
coincidentally discovered that walking became easier and
easier and that she could do a full day's walking and keep
up with her boyfriend without undue fatigue.

Swimming is another area to which Alexander
exponents have applied the Technique. Tony Buzan, who
lectures internationally on how to use your brain better,
is also an experienced long distance swimmer. When he
learnt the Technique it changed the way he swam. Instead
of fighting the water his strokes were smoother and more
effective. In particular giving the directions allowed him
to move his head much more easily for breathing and
the breathing itself became easier and fuller.

ELAINE IS SHORT AND HER BOYFRIEND IS TALL. THEY BOTH LIKE FELL-WALKING BUT SHE COULD NOT KEEP UP WITH HIM.

LIFTING AND CARRYING

We cannot avoid lifting and carrying, but we can avoid some of their harmful effects. In the course of lessons you will almost certainly be taught the position of mechanical advantage, or as we call it, monkey. Learning this position (or more accurately movement) gives you a chance to apply the Technique to any situation requiring power. It is the position humans naturally go into when they get ready to do something needing effort. Tennis players waiting to receive a serve, runners at the start of a race, golfers and batsmen in cricket are just some examples. It is seen most often in daily life when someone gets ready to lift an object.

The problem once again is habit. The solution once again is observation, inhibition and direction. This can be demonstrated by the difference between the habitual and the directed use of the body in lifting. In most people (habitual use) the spine is distorted, the body weight is too far forward and the muscles are overtensed. In

93

directed use the spine maintains its natural form, the body weight is far enough back to aid the lift and the muscles are released and free to stretch giving a springy elastic start to the movement.

WRITING

Often, it is when a person is writing that some of the most peculiar ways of treating a body can be seen. This, in turn, causes a corresponding clutch of problems, including neck pain, frozen shoulders, writer's cramp, headaches, back pain, stomach pain and so on. Looking at the way people write, it is not really surprising. The neck is often held very tense, shoulders are lifted, people lean heavily on one elbow, they tighten the wrist and fingers so that they become white. The legs are often twisted over each other and the feet lifted off the ground or tapping up and down almost as though the person was wanting to run away. All of these nervous reactions can be prevented and the result is not only the end of the pain, but much better handwriting and increased pleasure in the task.

The overall solution to these, and many other everyday problems, is not some slavishly mechanical use of the Technique. Teaching body mechanics or good posture will not solve the problems. I was told of the following by a leading expert on back pain when his team was asked to help a company to train its workers in lifting. They observed the workers and saw that they were trying to bend their backs and hold their legs straight when they lifted things. So, the team trained them in good body mechanics, that is, keeping the back straight and bending the knees to lift. The result was a reduction in the number of cases of back pain but an increase in the number of people having knee pain – a good example of not seeing the real causes because of not understanding the message of the Alexander Technique.

What is needed is a sensitive and personal re-education of the individual to help them see how they are reacting

OFTEN IT IS IN WRITING THAT WE SEE SOME OF THE MOST
PECULIAR WAYS OF TREATING OUR BODIES .

inappropriately to the demands placed on them and how
they can find a practical way of responding in a better
way.

REHABILITATION

One of the most important uses of the Technique is in
rehabilitation after an illness, injury or operation. During
this time the body is weak and needs the best possible
chance to re-build and repair itself by improved balance,
posture and movement. These, in addition to the usual
rehabilitation methods, help reduce mechanical forces
on damaged tissues and make recuperation a positive
possibility for a new and better approach to normal
life.

95

A BROADER PERSPECTIVE

Using Alexander lessons people from all kinds of backgrounds have learned how to improve their general levels of health and performance, as I hope I have shown in my examples. The Technique helps us to take a healthy interest in how we can improve the way we use ourselves. It teaches us how to see where we go wrong and the skill to do something about it. I find watching babies, wild animals, great sportsmen, dancers, and performing artists in general a great help in this. In this we see the most creative and powerful responses carried out with the greatest of skill in the face of enormous demands and stress.

The Technique penetrates to the centre of what we think being human is. It operates initially at the interface between what we call 'physical' and 'mental' or 'conscious' and 'subconscious'. In the longer term, by seeing the results of our conditioning and other environmental forces, we are faced with our ways of reacting to them and how we can prevent those reactions which are inappropriate. We are moving out of the fixed, subconscious and automatic towards a more conscious and flexible way of behaving. Although difficult to sustain at first, it becomes easier to the extent that it can be almost automatic but subject to choice. In short by developing conscious attention we become more able to choose and so deal with habits.

Too often we find ourselves stuck in a particular way of behaving based on fixed beliefs or fear. On the other hand 'changing' can be just as rigid a habit. It can be that the changes are just other ways of doing things badly and are an avoidance of the responsibility for making choices. In Alexander's own words, 'this work is about making choices and sticking to them against the habits of a lifetime.'

Because *we ourselves* are the instrument we must use, whatever we are doing, we need to know how to use ourselves well. As we develop this practical skill we are offered several possibilities. Firstly we gain in skill and health as has been shown. Additionally we can be more discriminating in our choice of activities as we have developed objective criteria for assessing whether or not they are actually beneficial. Thirdly we are able to develop the kind of dynamic constancy that is characteristic of well functioning natural systems. This gives the possibility of a more sensitive and constructive way of being which combines intelligence, flexibility, strength – and a good sense of humour! Through this we are given the opportunity to evaluate what we really want and how we want to behave. We then have the choice of working consciously with our own evolution, both inner and outèr, with the tools Alexander has provided.

So far I have talked about the Technique in relation to ourselves but the implications of the Technique go far beyond this. Unbalanced and destructive behaviours caused by end gaining are to be seen in personal relationships, how we treat our children, medical care, education, politics, business and international affairs to name but a few. Perhaps it is clearest in the way we treat nature. In all these cases our old, blind, instinctive – or more accurately, habitual – ways of treating ourselves, other people and the planet are creating more and more difficult problems.

Alexander's discovery of what we do to ourselves and how to stop doing it, so we can perform whatever we do well, whilst preserving our health and sanity can, in my view, be extended to all these vital areas. By following Alexander's approach, we have the possibility of improving not just our individual state, but that of the world.

USEFUL
ADDRESSES

Further information and a list of qualified teachers of
the Alexander Technique can be obtained from the
following addresses. Please enclose a large stamped
addressed envelope with your enquiry.

UNITED KINGDOM

Society of Teachers of the Alexander Technique (STAT)
10 London House
266 Fulham Road
London SW10 9EL

Alexander Research Trust
18 Lansdowne Road
London W11 3LL

CANADA

Canadian Society of Teachers of the Alexander Technique
(CANSTAT)
460 Palmerston Boulevard
Toronto
Ontario
P7A 4A2

AUSTRALIA

Australian Society of Teachers of the Alexander
Technique (AUSTAT)
PO Box 529
Milsons Point
Sydney 2061
New South Wales

DENMARK

International School for the FM Alexander Technique
J. Berthelsensv. 15A
9400 Nørresundby

FURTHER READING

The Alexander Principle, Dr Wilfred Barlow (pub: Gollancz, 1973)

More Talk of Alexander, Dr Wilfred Barlow (pub: Gollancz, 1978)

The Use of the Self, F M Alexander (pub: latest edition, Gollancz, 1986)

The Constructive Conscious Control of the Individual, F M Alexander (pub: latest edition, Centerline Press, 1984)

The Man Who Mistook his Wife for a Hat, Oliver Sacks (pub: Paladin, 1986)

'Form and Function of the Erect Human Spine' in *Orthopaedics and Related Research*, volume 25, pages 55–63. E Asmussen and K Klausen (pub: 1963)

'Alignment of the Human Body in Standing' in the *European Journal of Applied Physiology*, pages 109–115, A M Woodhull et al (pub: 1985)

'Lumbar disc pressure and myoelectric back muscle activity during sitting', *Scandanavian Journal of Rehabilitation Medicine*, volume 6, pages 104–114, B J Andersson et al (pub: 1974)

The Cause of Lumbar Back Pain, John Gorman (pub: John Gorman, 1984)

Yoga in the 'Know the Game' series, Chris Stevens (pub: A & C Black, 1985)

The Endeavour of Jean Fernel, Sir Charles Sherrington (pub: Cambridge University Press, 1946)

Body Awareness in Action, Professor F P Jones (pub: latest edition, Schocken, 1979)

Body Learning, Michael Gelb (pub: Aurum Press, 1981)

Medical and Physiological Aspects of the Alexander Technique, Chris Stevens (editor) (pub: Alexander Research Press, 1988)

INDEX

ABOUT THE AUTHOR

CHRIS STEVENS, BEd, MSTAT, is an experienced teacher of the Alexander Technique. He works in Denmark, where he also directs the training of future Alexander Technique teachers, in Aalborg.

He has published several research papers, based on his scientific studies of the Alexander Technique at the Universities of London and Copenhagen. This is his second book.